THE ULTIMATE VEGAN SIDE DISHES COOKBOOK

50 vibrant, kitchen-tested recipes of delicious side dishes

Laura Mckinney

the reader will render any resulting actions solely under their purview. There are no scenarios in which the publisher or the original author of this work can be in any fashion deemed liable for any hardship or damages that may befall them after undertaking information described herein.
Additionally, the information in the following pages is intended only for informational purposes and should thus be thought of as universal. As befitting its nature, it is presented without assurance regarding its prolonged validity or interim quality. Trademarks that are mentioned are done without written consent and can in no way be considered an endorsement from the trademark holder.

Table of contents

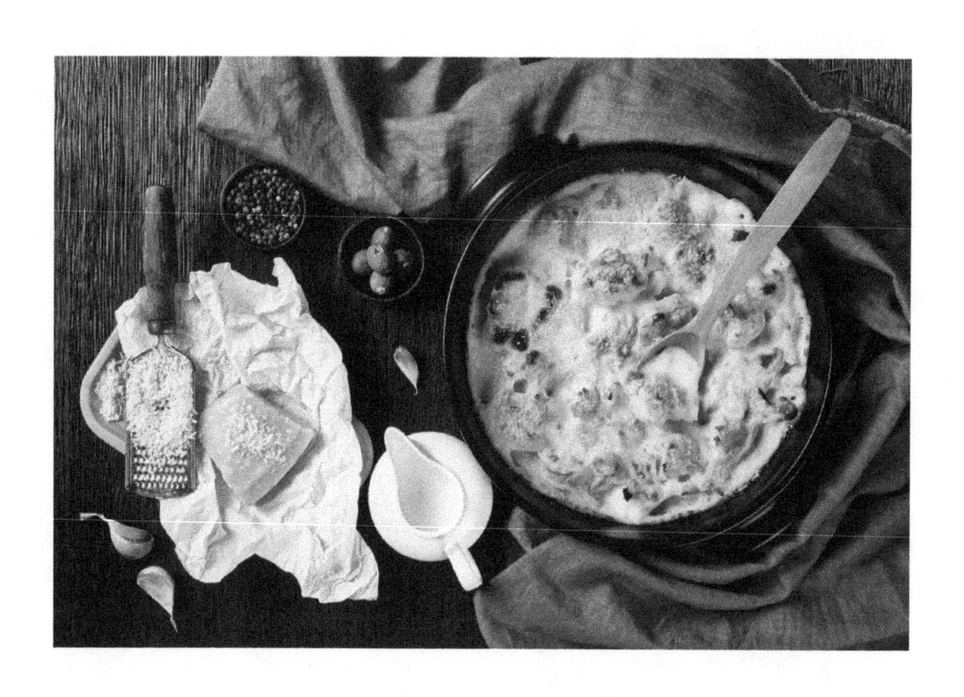

Introduction

Veganism is one of the most followed trends around the world today.
There are many people who have decided not to take more food products deriving from animal products and to follow a lifestyle in harmony with nature. The history of the vegan diet began in 1944 with a diet specially formulated for the purpose, five years later Leslie J Cross suggested the idea of veganism by supporting the idea of emancipating animals from human exploitation.
Over the years, veganism has become not only a food habit but a real lifestyle, influencing hundreds of thousands of people, for whom it shares an attitude of respect and protection of animals and nature in general.

Veganism involves the abolition of the diet of any food derived from meat, poultry, seafood, and dairy products. Contrary to what one might think, however, the vegan diet is very varied and full of succulent and very different dishes, to satisfy any preference. From breakfast to dinner you can vary to your liking with very good and satisfying sweet and savory dishes. The only condition is that each meal is made with ingredients of plant origin. And don't think that the vegan diet has limits on nutrients, because vitamins, minerals, and vital proteins can be taken from vegetables, fruits, cereals, nuts, and seeds. It will be enough to practice a little and the result will certainly be in line with our expectations, thanks also to an increasingly refined technology of cooking meals. Vegan food is very varied, from vegan ice cream, to burritos, cheese, burgers, mayonnaise and so much more. Being vegan does not mean depriving yourself of something, on the contrary, it means improving your lifestyle in harmony with the nature of which we are part.

The vegan diet also includes the consumption of lettuce, pasta, chips, bread, and various sauces.

The reasons that push people to become vague can be the most disparate, the lifestyle they assume certainly benefits everyone! The vegetable diet is sufficiently rich in iron, folic acid, magnesium, vitamins C and B1 which are essential for our body. At the same time, the vegan diet can never include a high amount of saturated fat and cholesterol.

Also, veganism has obvious health benefits, helping to prevent serious diseases such as stroke, type 2 diabetes, obesity, colon and prostate cancer, hypertension, and ischemic heart disease. There are no age preclusions to follow a vegan diet, however, we recommend greater attention to the daily meal ratio, to avoid nutritional deficiencies.

In this cookbook, you will find 50 delicious recipes that will make you want to get up in the morning. There are recipes for every taste, just follow our advice and you can make real culinary masterpieces. Forget the boredom of thinking about what to eat, this cookbook will give you the right inspiration.

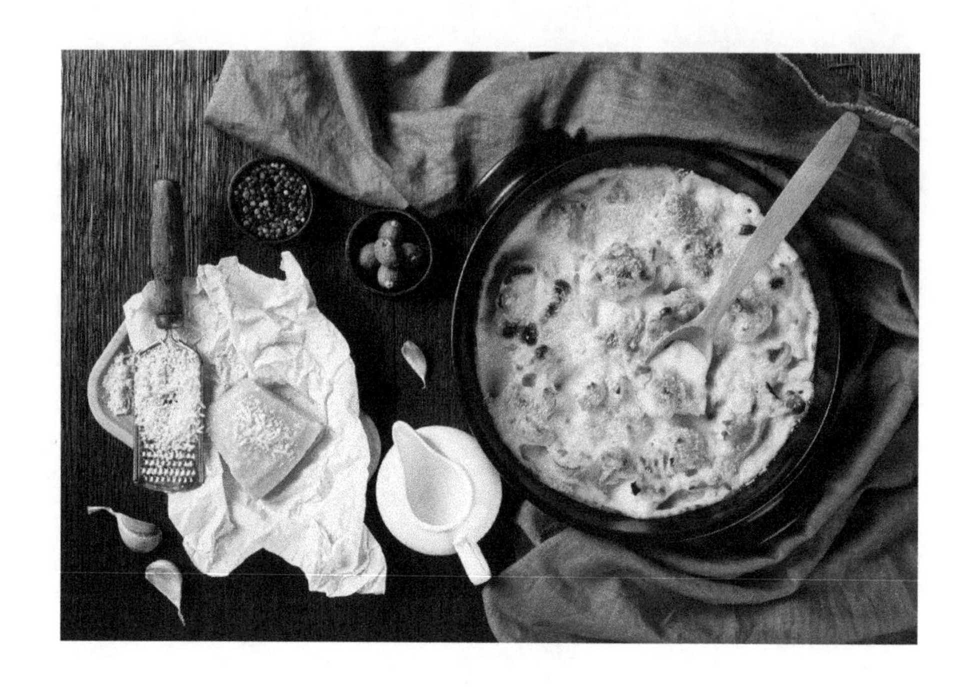

Glazed Bok Choy

Prep time: 15 minutes Cooking time: 4 minutes Servings: 4

Ingredients:

- 1-pound bok choy
- 1 tablespoon Maple syrup
- 1 tablespoon sesame oil
- 1 teaspoon ground cumin
- ½ teaspoon minced garlic
- 1 teaspoon ground ginger
- 1 tablespoon apple cider vinegar
- 1 tablespoon sesame seeds
- ½ cup of water

Directions:

1. Chop bok choy roughly and sprinkle with maple syrup, ground cumin, sesame oil, minced garlic, ground ginger, and apple cider vinegar.
2. Mix up the vegetables and let them marinade for 10 minutes.
3. Transfer the bok choy and all the liquid in the instant pot. Add water and cook on Manual mode (High pressure) for 4 minutes.

4. Then make quick pressure release.
5. Transfer the cooked bok choy in the serving bowls and sprinkle with sesame seeds.

Nutrition value/serving: calories 76, fat 4.9, fiber 1.5, carbs 7.1, protein 2.3

Pumpkin Puree

Prep time: 15 minutes Cooking time: 15 minutes Servings: 6

Ingredients:

- 2-pound pumpkin, peeled, chopped
- 1/3 cup almond milk
- 1 cup of water
- 1 teaspoon dried oregano

Directions:

1. Put chopped pumpkin in the instant pot. Add water and close the lid.
2. Cook on Manual mode (High pressure) for 15 minutes. Use natural pressure release for 10 minutes.
3. Strain pumpkin and transfer it in the food processor.
4. Add almond milk and dried oregano. Blend the mixture until smooth.
5. The pumpkin puree should be served only warm.

Nutrition value/serving: calories 83, fat 3.6, fiber 4.8, carbs 13.1, protein 2

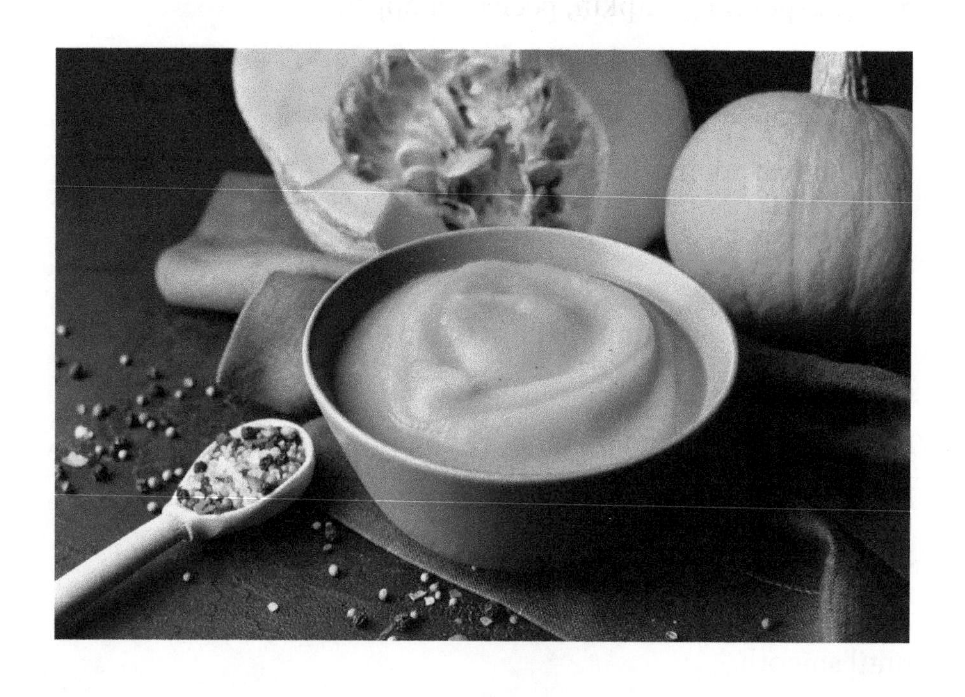

Lemon Potatoes

Prep time: 7 minutes Cooking time: 8 minutes Servings: 4

Ingredients:

- 4 white potatoes
- 1 teaspoon lemon zest
- 1 teaspoon Pink salt
- 1 tablespoon fresh dill, chopped
- 1 teaspoon dried oregano
- 2 tablespoon lemon juice
- ¼ cup vegetable broth
- 1 tablespoon olive oil

Directions:

1. Wash potatoes carefully and chop roughly.
2. Whisk together lemon juice, olive oil, dried oregano, and fresh dill.
3. Pour olive oil mixture over the potatoes and sprinkle with salt. Shake well and transfer in the instant pot.
4. Add vegetable broth and cook on Manual mode for 8 minutes.
5. Allow natural pressure release.

Nutrition value/serving: calories 185, fat 3.9, fiber 5.4, carbs 34.5, protein 4.2

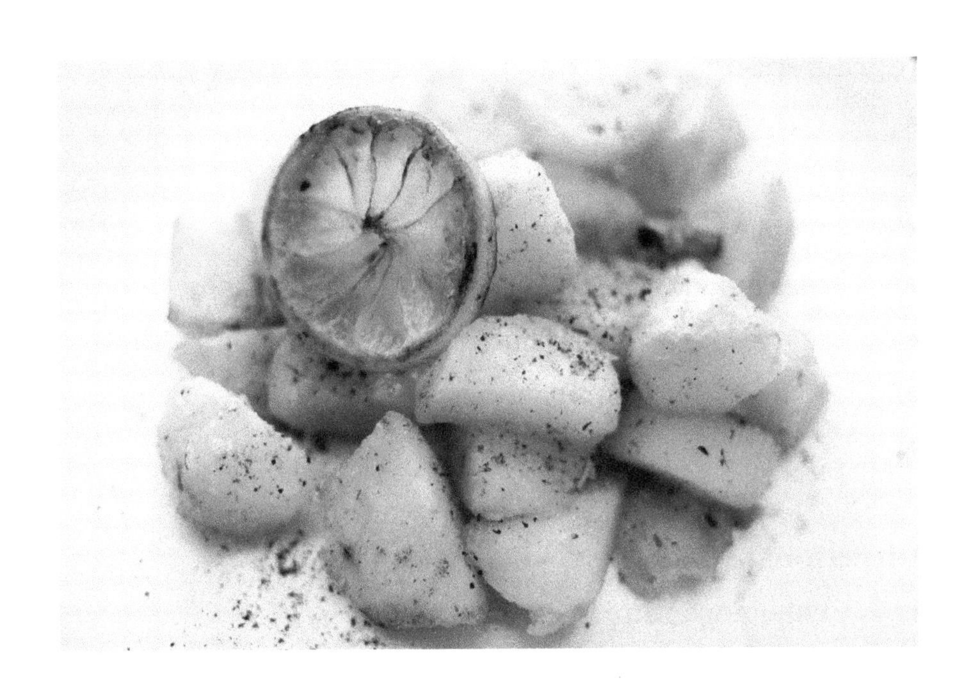

Quinoa with Basil and Lemongrass

Prep time: 15 minutes Cooking time: 3 minutes Servings: .3

Ingredients:

- 1 cup quinoa
- 1 cup vegetable broth
- 1 tablespoon lemongrass, chopped
- 1 teaspoon dried basil
- 1 tablespoon almond butter
- ¾ teaspoon ground nutmeg
- 1/3 teaspoon Pink salt

Directions:

1. Put quinoa in an instant pot.
2. Add vegetable broth, ground nutmeg, and salt. Close the lid, seal it, and set Manual mode (high pressure).
3. Cook quinoa for 3 minutes and allow natural pressure release for 10 minutes.
4. In the cooked quinoa add almond butter, lemongrass and dried basil. Mix the side dish up.
5. The side dish is cooked.

Nutrition value/serving: calories 259, fat 7.1, fiber 4.6, carbs 38.4, protein 10.8

Tender Yellow Couscous

Prep time: 15 minutes Cooking time: 5 minutes Servings: 4

Ingredients:

- 1 ½ cup yellow couscous
- 2 cups of water
- 1 tablespoon olive oil
- 1 teaspoon salt

Directions:

1. Preheat instant pot on Saute mode for 3 minutes.
2. Pour olive oil inside it and add couscous.
3. Stir it gently and saute for 2 minutes.
4. Then add water and salt. Close the lid. Set manual mode (High pressure).
5. Cook the side dish for 2 minutes.
6. Release the pressure manually for 10 minutes.

Nutrition value/serving: calories 96, fat 3.6, fiber 0.8, carbs 13.5, protein 2.2

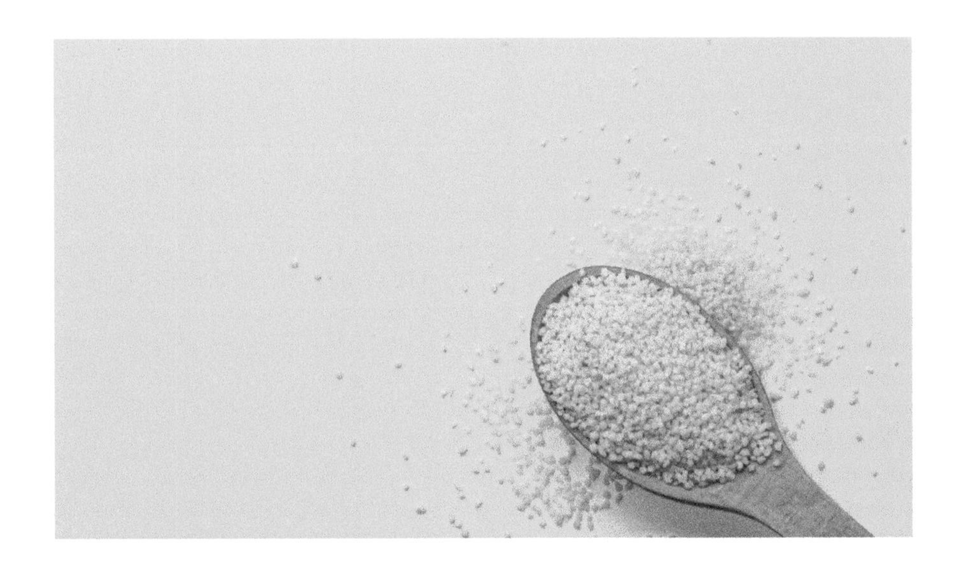

Mashed Potato

Prep time: 10 minutes Cooking time: 10 minutes Servings: 6

Ingredients:

- 6 potatoes, peeled, chopped
- 1 cup of water
- ¼ cup of coconut milk
- 1 tablespoon coconut yogurt
- 1 teaspoon salt
- 1 tablespoon chives, chopped

Directions:

1. Place potato and water in the instant pot. Add salt and close the lid.
2. Cook the vegetables on Manual mode for 10 minutes.
3. Then use quick pressure release.
4. Open the lid, drain water from the potatoes and mash them.
5. Add coconut yogurt, coconut milk, and chopped chives.
6. Mix it up until soft and smooth.

Nutrition value/serving: calories 171, fat 2.6, fiber 5.3, carbs 34.2, protein 3.9

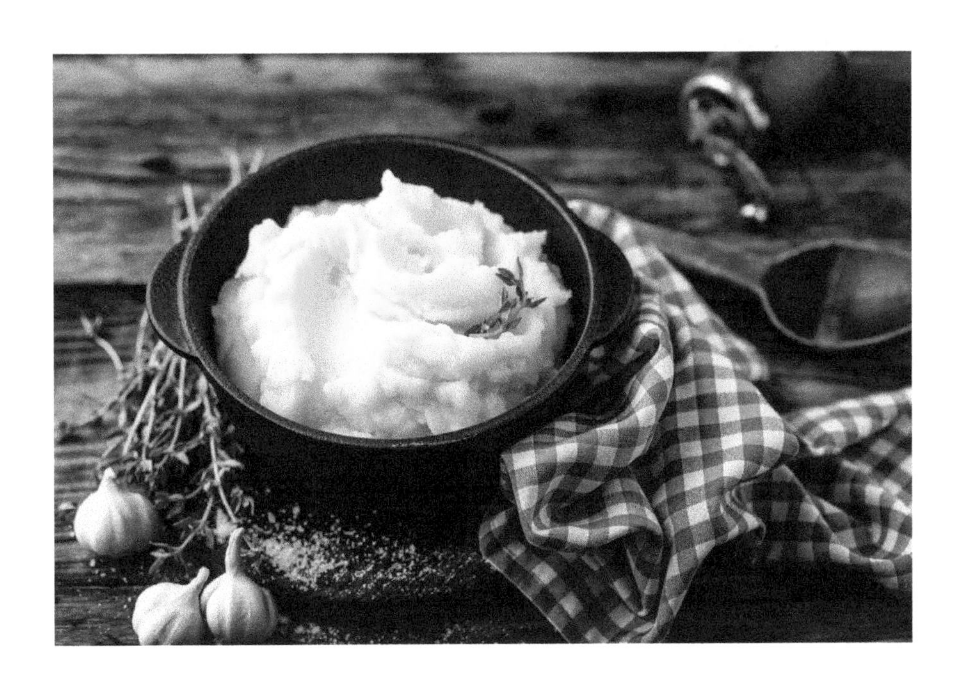

Vermicelli Bowl

Prep time: 10 minutes Cooking time: 6 minutes Servings: 2

Ingredients:

- 1 cup vermicelli, roasted
- ½ yellow onion, diced
- ½ jalapeno pepper, chopped
- 1 cup of water
- 1 teaspoon ground cumin
- ¼ teaspoon ground coriander
- 1 teaspoon dried rosemary
- 1 teaspoon ground ginger
- 2 red bell peppers, chopped
- 1 teaspoon olive oil

Directions:

1. Put diced onion, jalapeno pepper, ground cumin, coriander, rosemary, ginger, and bell peppers in the instant pot.
2. Add olive oil, stir it and saute for 3 minutes.
3. Then add vermicelli and water. Close the lid and set manual mode (High pressure) for 3 minutes.
4. Make a quick pressure release.

5. Shake the meal with the help of fork gently and transfer into the bowls.

Nutrition value/serving: calories 184, fat 3.6, fiber 3.8, carbs 34.3, protein 5.3

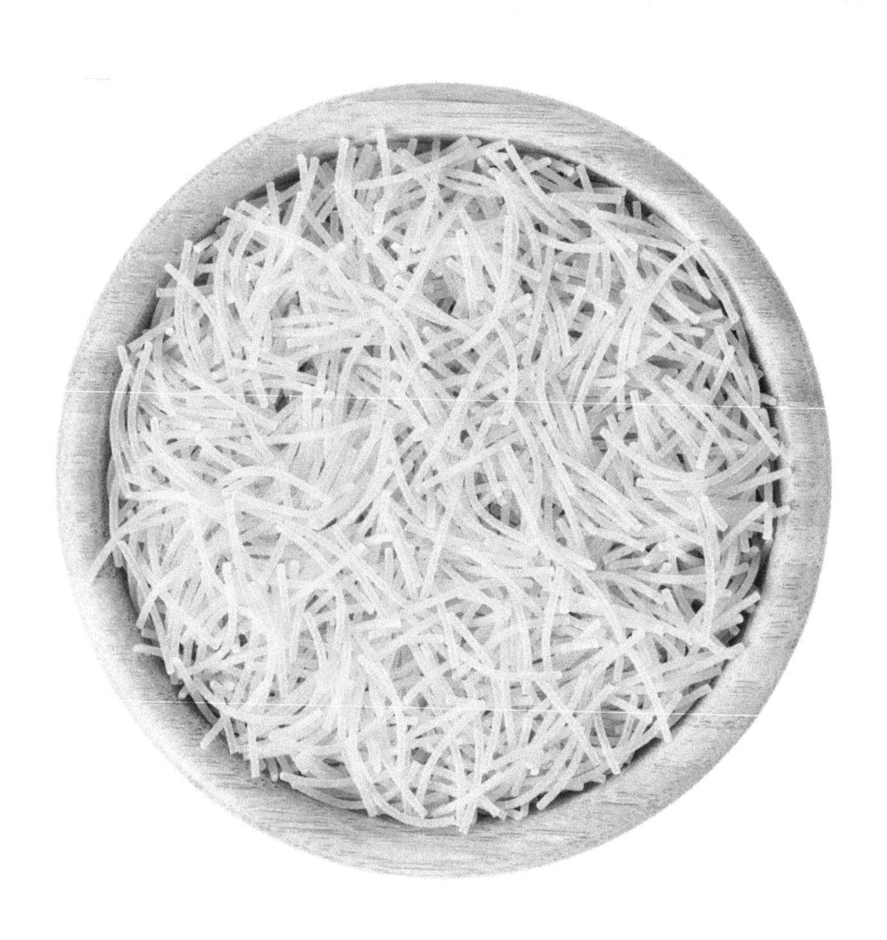

Broccoli Rice

Prep time: 10 minutes Cooking time: 1 minute Servings: 4

Ingredients:

- 2 ½ cup broccoli florets
- 1 teaspoon salt
- 1 teaspoon grinded peppercorn
- ½ cup of water
- 1 teaspoon olive oil
- 1 teaspoon minced garlic

Directions:

1. Put broccoli florets in the food processor and blend until you get broccoli rice.
2. Pour water in the instant pot.
3. Then place broccoli rice in the instant pot pan.
4. Add peppercorns, salt, olive oil, and minced garlic. Mix up the ingredients.
5. Transfer the pan in the instant pot and close the lid.
6. Set manual mode and cook on High for 1 minute. Make a quick pressure release.
7. Chill the cauliflower rice for 2-5 minutes before serving.

Nutrition value/serving: calories 32, fat 1.4, fiber 1.6, carbs 4.4, protein 1.7

Sweet Potato Mash

Prep time: 10 minutes Cooking time: 9 minutes Servings: 6

Ingredients:

- 2 cups sweet potatoes, peeled, chopped
- 1 teaspoon salt
- 1 teaspoon ground black pepper
- 1 cup vegetable broth
- 1 tablespoon fresh parsley, chopped

Directions:

1. Put potatoes, salt, and vegetable broth in the instant pot.
2. Close the lid and set manual mode. Cook on High for 9 minutes.
3. Then make quick pressure release, strain the sweet potatoes and mash until smooth.
4. Add chopped parsley and ground black pepper in the mashed sweet potato. Mix up well.

Nutrition value/serving: calories 67, fat 0.3, fiber 2.2, carbs 14.4, protein 1.6

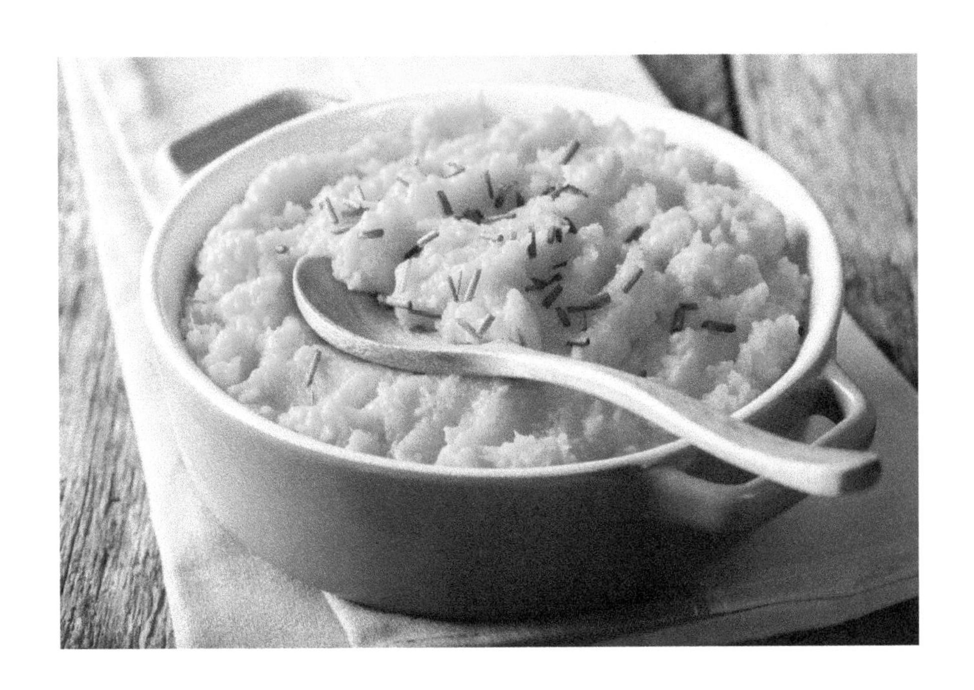

Red Cabbage with Apples

Prep time: 10 minutes Cooking time: 7 minutes Servings: 3

Ingredients:

- 1-pound red cabbage
- 1 apple, chopped
- 1 teaspoon salt
- ¼ cup of coconut milk
- ¾ cup almond milk
- ½ teaspoon chili flakes

Directions:

1. Shred red cabbage and mix it up with salt.
2. Transfer the mixture in the instant pot. Add coconut milk, almond milk, and chili flakes.
3. Then add apple and set manual mode (High pressure).
4. Cook the cabbage for 7 minutes. Then allow natural pressure release.
5. Transfer the meal into the serving bowls and mix up well before serving.

Nutrition value/serving: calories 123, fat 5.1, fiber 6, carbs 20.2, protein 2.6

Garlic Spaghetti Squash

Prep time: 15 minutes Cooking time: 10 minutes Servings: 4

Ingredients:

- 1 teaspoon minced garlic
- 1 teaspoon onion powder
- ½ teaspoon chili flakes
- 1 teaspoon apple cider vinegar
- 1-pound spaghetti squash, halved, seeds removed
- 1 tablespoon Italian seasoning
- 1 cup water, for cooking

Directions:

1. Pour water in the instant pot and insert steamer rack.
2. Arrange spaghetti squash on the rack and close the lid.
3. Cook it on High for 10 minutes. Then allow natural pressure release for 5 minutes.
4. Check if the spaghetti squash is soft and shred the flesh with the help of a fork.
5. Put the squash shred in the bowl.

6. For serving the squash, add onion powder, minced garlic, chili flakes, apple cider vinegar, and Italian seasoning. Mix it up.

Nutrition value/serving: calories 49, fat 1.7, fiber 0, carbs 9, protein 0.8

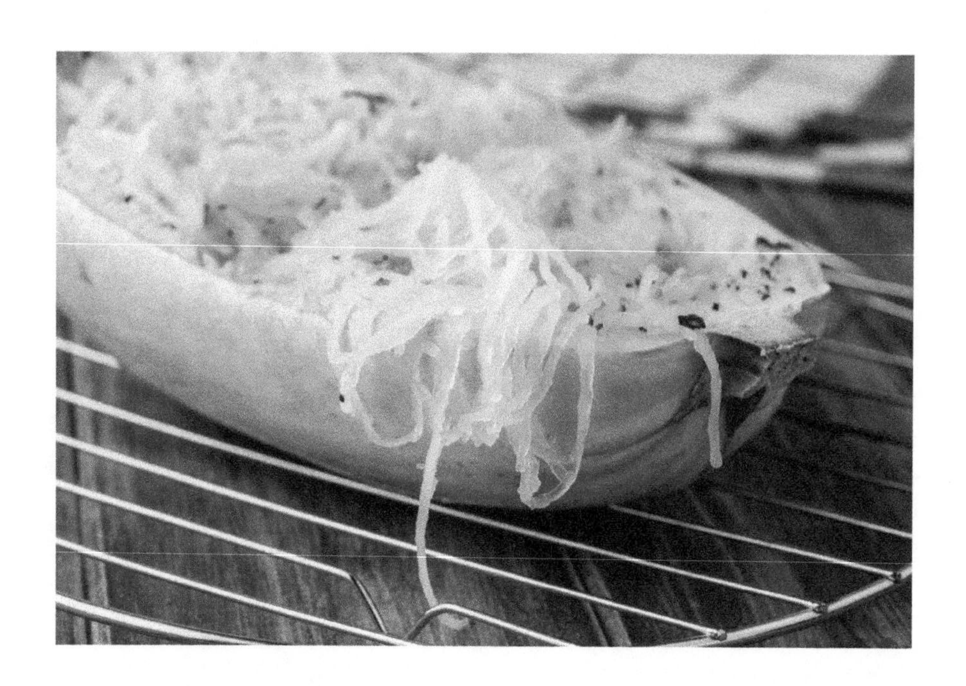

Baked Potato

Prep time: 10 minutes Cooking time: 11 minutes Servings: 2

Ingredients:

- 2 potatoes
- 2 teaspoons vegan mayonnaise
- 1 teaspoon chives, chopped
- ½ cup of water

Directions:

1. Pour water in the instant pot and insert steamer rack.
2. Put potatoes on the rack and close the lid.
3. Set Manual mode (High pressure) and cook for 11 minutes. Then use quick pressure release.
4. Transfer the potatoes on the plate and cut into halves.
5. Sprinkle them with mayonnaise and chives.

Nutrition value/serving: calories 159, fat 1.4, fiber 5.1, carbs 33.8, protein 3.6

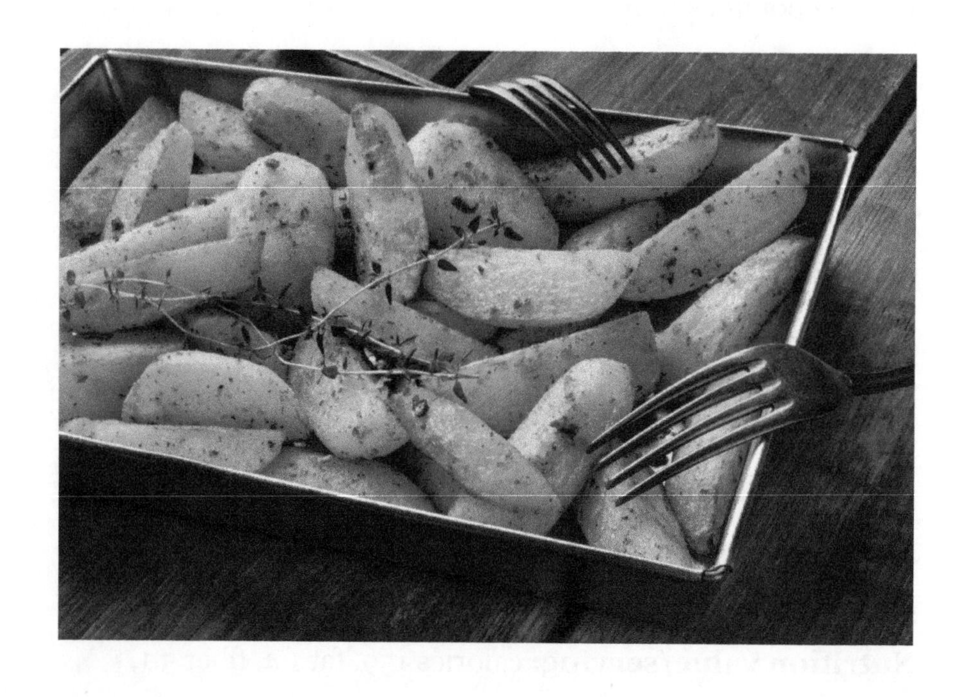

Vegan Applesauce

Prep time: 10 minutes Cooking time: 10 minutes Servings: 4

Ingredients:

- 5 apples
- 1/3 cup water
- 1 teaspoon ground cinnamon
- ¼ teaspoon vanilla extract

Directions:

1. Peel the apples and remove seeds.
2. Put apples in the instant pot and sprinkle with ground cinnamon, vanilla extract, and water.
3. Close the lid and cook on Manual mode (High pressure) for 10 minutes.
4. After this, use quick pressure release.
5. Transfer the mixture in the blender and blend until smooth.
6. Place applesauce in the glass jar and let it rest in the fridge for 30 minutes before serving.

Nutrition value/serving: calories 147, fat 0.5, fiber 7.1, carbs 39, protein 0.8

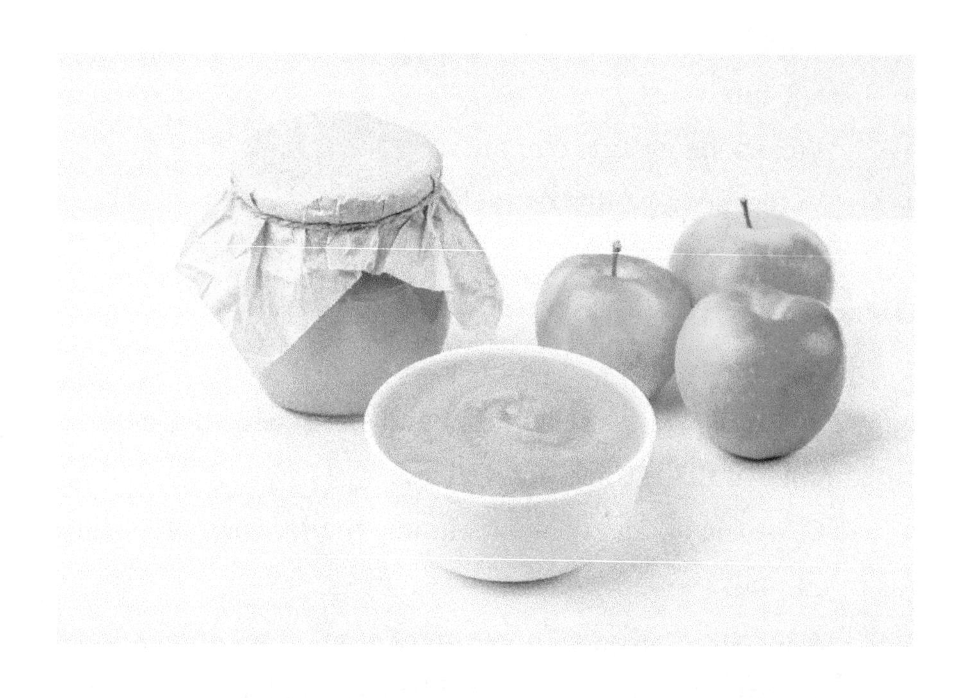

Mexican Rice

Prep time: 10 minutes Cooking time: 8 minutes Servings: 4

Ingredients:

- 1 cup long grain rice
- 1 tablespoon tomato paste
- ¼ cup corn kernels, canned
- 1 teaspoon smoked paprika
- 1 teaspoon chili flakes
- 1 teaspoon salt
- 2 cups vegetable broth
- 1 carrot, chopped
- 2 tablespoons olive oil

1. Pour olive oil in the instant pot and set Saute mode.
2. Add rice and start to cook it.
3. Add chili flakes, salt, and ¼ cup of vegetable broth. Stir it.
4. Add tomato paste and stir until rice gets the red color.
5. Then add corn kernels, smoked paprika, carrot, and all remaining vegetable broth.
6. Set Manual mode (High pressure) and close the lid. Seal it.

7. Cook rice for 4 minutes. Use quick pressure release.

Nutrition value/serving: calories 267, fat 8.2, fiber 1.6, carbs 41.8, protein 6.4

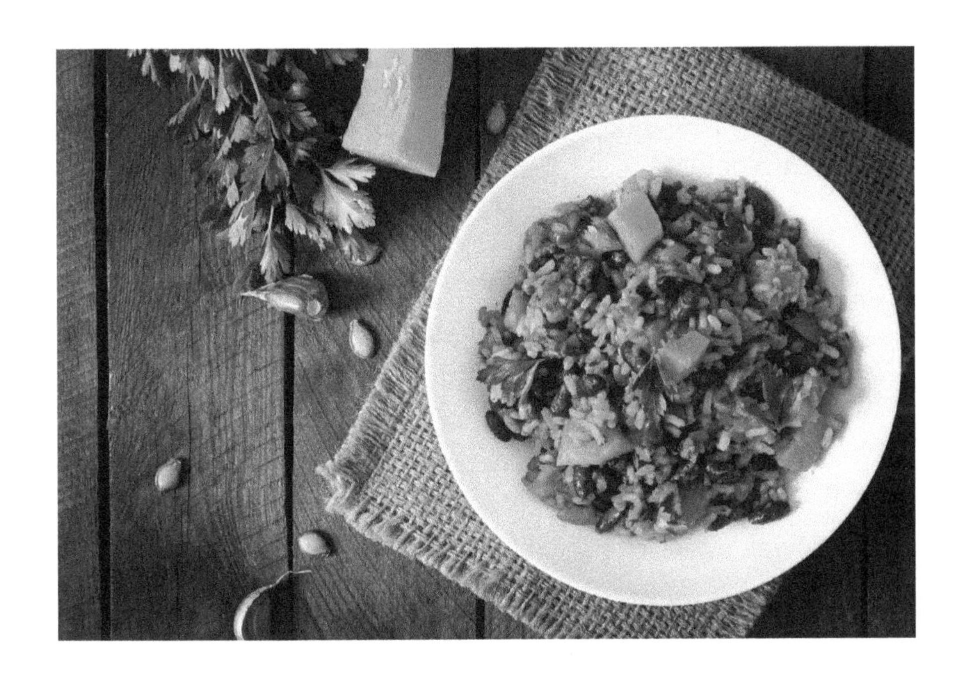

Polenta

Prep time: 5 minutes Cooking time: 8 minutes Servings: 5

Ingredients:

- 1 cup polenta
- 4 cups vegetable broth
- 2 tablespoons coconut milk
- ½ teaspoon ground black pepper
- 1 teaspoon salt

Directions:

1. Whisk together polenta and vegetable broth.
2. Pour mixture in the instant pot. Add salt.
3. Close the lid and cook it on Manual mode (High pressure) for 8 minutes. Use quick pressure release/
4. Transfer cooked polenta in the bowl and stir well. You need to get the creamy texture of the meal.
5. Add ground black pepper and coconut milk. Stir it before serving.

Nutrition value/serving: calories 156, fat 2.8, fiber 1, carbs 25.5, protein 6.3

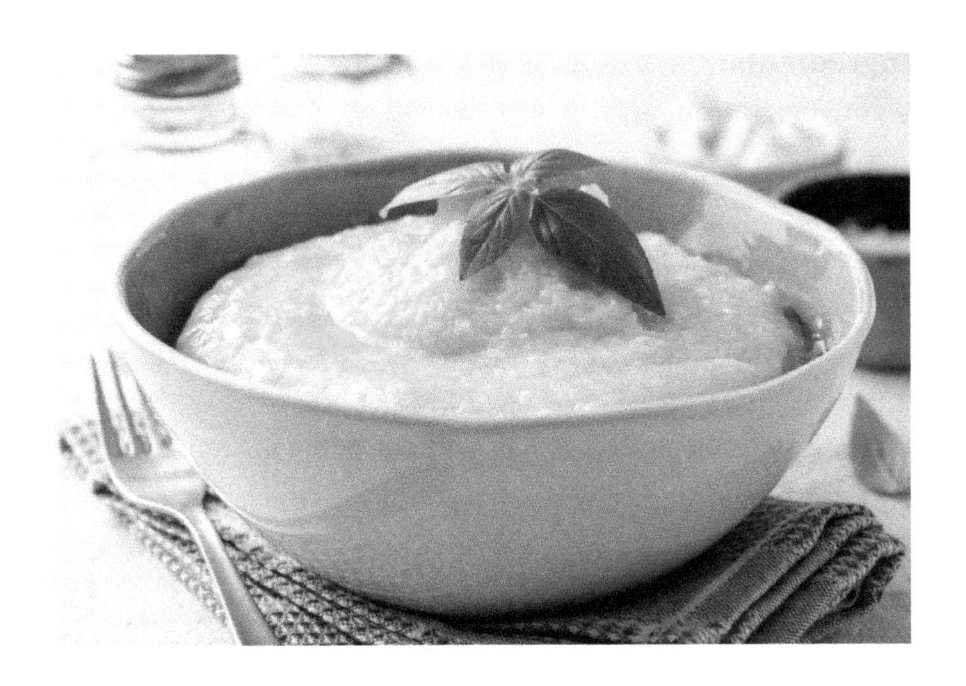

Pasta Marinara

Prep time: 5 minutes Cooking time: 5 minutes Servings: 4

Ingredients:

- 13 oz spaghetti
- 1 cup marinara sauce
- ½ cup of water
- 1 teaspoon dried basil

Directions:

1. Break spaghetti into half and put in the instant pot.
2. Add marinara sauce and water. Close the lid.
3. Seal it and cook on Manual mode (high pressure) for 5 minutes.
4. Make a quick pressure release.
5. Transfer cooked pasta in the bowl and sprinkle with dried basil.

Nutrition value/serving: calories 320, fat 3.8, fiber 1.6, carbs 59, protein 11.5

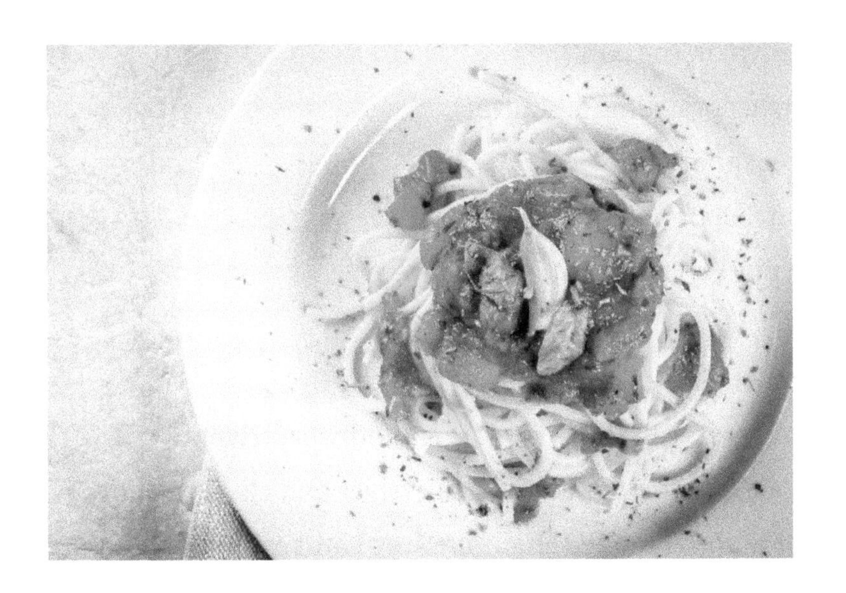

Butter Corn

Prep time: 5 minutes Cooking time: 2 minutes Servings: 4

Ingredients:

- 4 corn on the cob
- 4 teaspoon almond butter
- 1 teaspoon salt
- ½ teaspoon minced garlic
- ½ cup of water

Directions:

1. Pour water in the instant pot and insert trivet.
2. Place corn on the cobs on the trivet and close the lid.
3. Set manual mode (High pressure) and cook for 2 minutes.
4. Use natural pressure release.
5. Churn together almond butter, salt, and minced garlic.
6. Spread the corn on the cobs with the churned mixture before serving.

Nutrition value/serving: calories 229, fat 9, fiber 3.5, carbs 34.7, protein 8.1

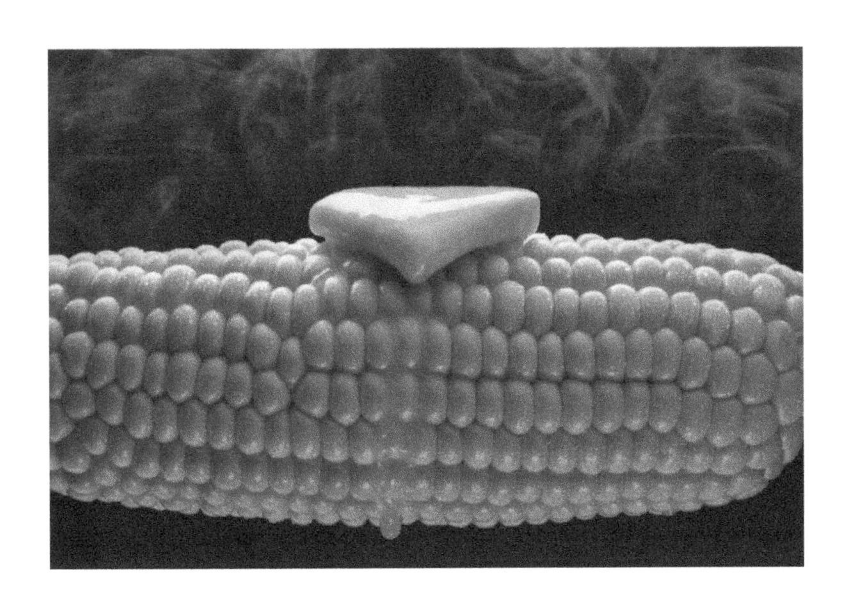

Artichoke Petals

Prep time: 5 minutes Cooking time: 7 minutes Servings: 4

Ingredients:

- 1-pound artichoke petals
- 1 teaspoon salt
- ½ cup of coconut milk

Directions:

1. Place artichoke petals, salt, and coconut milk in the instant pot.
2. Close the lid and set Manual mode.
3. Cook on High pressure for 7 minutes. Then allow natural pressure release for 5 minutes.
4. Mix up the vegetables before serving.

Nutrition value/serving: calories 122, fat 7.3, fiber 6.8, carbs 13.6, protein 4.4

Beets

Prep time: 10 minutes Cooking time: 17 minutes Servings: 4

Ingredients:

- 2-pound beets, peeled
- 1 teaspoon ground black pepper
- 1 tablespoon olive oil
- 1 cup water, for cooking

Directions:

1. Cut the bets into the medium cubes.
2. Pour water in the instant pot and insert trivet.
3. Place beets on the trivet and close the lid.
4. Cook the meal for 17 minutes on Manual mode (High pressure). Then use quick pressure.
5. Transfer beets in the bowl and sprinkle with ground black pepper and olive oil before serving.

Nutrition value/serving: calories 131, fat 3.9, fiber 4.7, carbs 22.9, protein 3.9

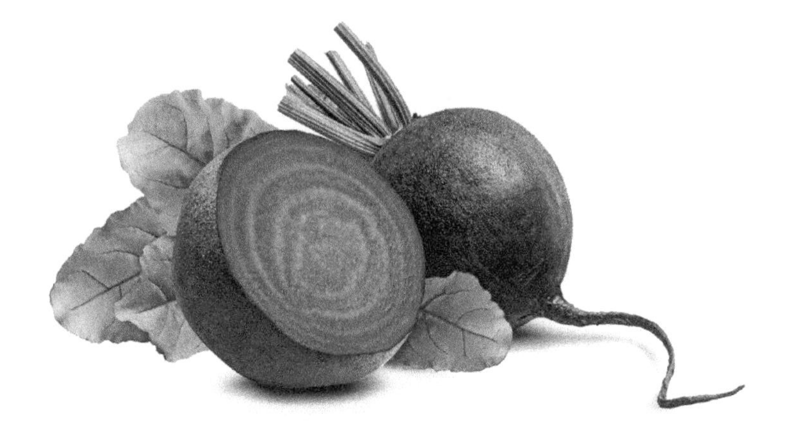

Tender Sweet Peppers

Prep time: 10 minutes Cooking time: 13 minutes Servings: 4

Ingredients:

- 2 red sweet peppers
- 1 green bell pepper
- 1 yellow sweet pepper
- 1 garlic clove, peeled
- 1 tomato, chopped
- ¼ cup fresh dill, chopped
- 2 tablespoons sesame oil
- ½ cup of water

Directions:

1. Trim the peppers and cut into the strips.
2. Preheat instant pot on Saute mode.
3. Add olive oil, garlic clove, and chopped tomato.
4. Saute the ingredients for 3 minutes. Mix up.
5. Add pepper strips and add water.
6. Close the lid and cook on Saute mode for 10 minutes.
7. When the peppers are tender – they are cooked. Don't cook a long time to avoid overcooking.

Nutrition value/serving: calories 110, fat 7.3, fiber 2.2, carbs 11.5, protein 2

Spiced Okra

Prep time: 10 minutes Cooking time: 22 minutes Servings: 5

Ingredients:

- 1-pound okra
- 1 teaspoon salt
- ½ teaspoon chili flakes
- ½ teaspoon cayenne pepper
- 1 teaspoon red chili pepper
- ½ cup of water
- 1 teaspoon almond butter

Directions:

1. Preheat instant pot on Saute mode for 2 minutes and place almond butter.
2. Meanwhile, slice okra.
3. Transfer it in the instant pot and sprinkle with chili flakes, salt, and red chili pepper.
4. Add water and mix up gently.
5. Close the lid and saute the vegetables for 20 minutes.
6. Mix up the okra before serving.

Nutrition value/serving: calories 57, fat 2, fiber 3.3, carbs 7.6, protein 2.5

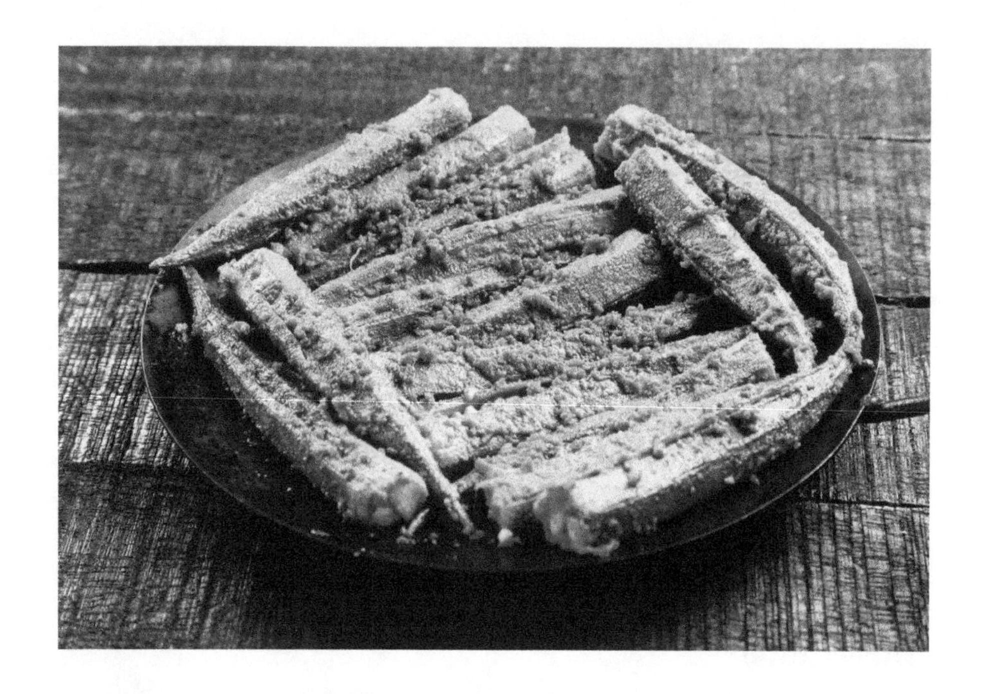

Sweet Baby Carrots

Prep time: 5 minutes Cooking time: 3 minutes Servings: 2

Ingredients:

- 1 cup baby carrots
- 1 tablespoon honey
- 1 teaspoon ground cinnamon
- ¼ teaspoon pumpkin spices
- 1 teaspoon coconut oil
- ¼ cup of water

Directions:

1. Mix up together water, honey, ground cinnamon, and pumpkin spices.
2. Whisk the liquid and pour it in the instant pot.
3. Add baby carrots and coconut oil. Close the lid.
4. Cook the side dish for 3 minutes on Manual mode (High pressure). Use the quick pressure release.
5. Serve the cooked baby carrots with the sweet sauce from the instant pot.

Nutrition value/serving: calories 73, fat 2.3, fiber 2.2, carbs 13.7, protein 0.1

Soft Kale

Prep time: 10 minutes Cooking time: 3 minutes Servings: 2

Ingredients:

- 1 cup kale
- ½ cup of water
- 1 teaspoon almond butter
- ½ teaspoon salt

Directions:

1. Chop the kale roughly and place in the instant pot. Add water.
2. Close the lid and seal it.
3. Set Manual mode (high pressure) and cook kale for 3 minutes. Then allow natural pressure release.
4. Transfer the cooked kale in the bowls and sprinkle with salt and almond butter.
5. Mix it up before serving.

Nutrition value/serving: calories 66, fat 4.5, fiber 1.3, carbs 5, protein 2.7

Cauliflower Rice

Prep time: 10 minutes Cooking time: 12 minutes Servings: 4

Ingredients:

- 1 ½-pound cauliflower head
- 1 cup of water
- 1 teaspoon salt
- 1 tablespoon fresh dill, chopped
- 2 tablespoons almond yogurt

Directions:

1. Pour water in the instant pot and insert steamer rack.
2. Place cauliflower on the rack and close the lid. Seal it.
3. Set manual mode (high pressure) and cook cauliflower for 12 minutes. Then make quick pressure release.
4. Transfer cooked cauliflower in the big bowl. With the help of the potato masher mash it gently until you get cauliflower rice.
5. Add dill, salt, and almond yogurt. Mix it up.

Nutrition value/serving: calories 50, fat 0.5, fiber 4.4, carbs 10.1, protein 3.7

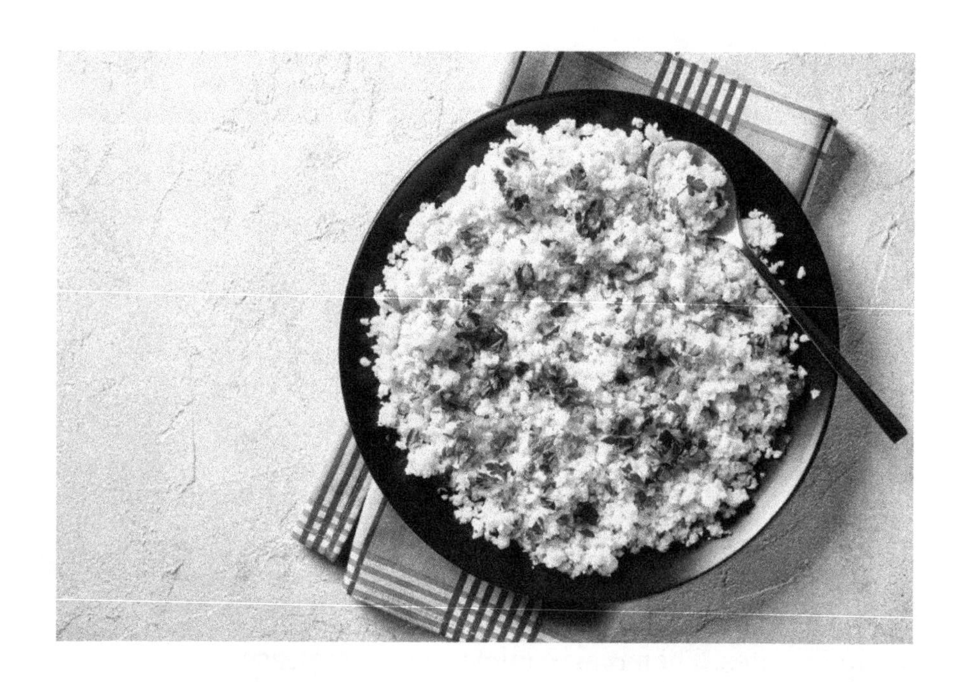

Barley

Prep time: 20 minutes Cooking time: 30 minutes Servings: 3

Ingredients:

- 1 cup barley
- 2 cups of water
- 1 teaspoon salt
- 1 tablespoon olive oil
- 1 teaspoon turmeric
- ½ teaspoon smoked paprika

Directions:

1. Set saute mode and pour olive oil in the instant pot.
2. Preheat it for 1-2 minutes and add barley. Stir it and cook for 3 minutes.
3. After this, add salt, turmeric, smoked paprika, and water.
4. Close the lid and switch on Manual mode (high pressure).
5. Cook barley for 25 minutes. Allow natural pressure release for 15 minutes.

Nutrition value/serving: calories 261, fat 6.2, fiber 10.9, carbs 45.7, protein 7.8

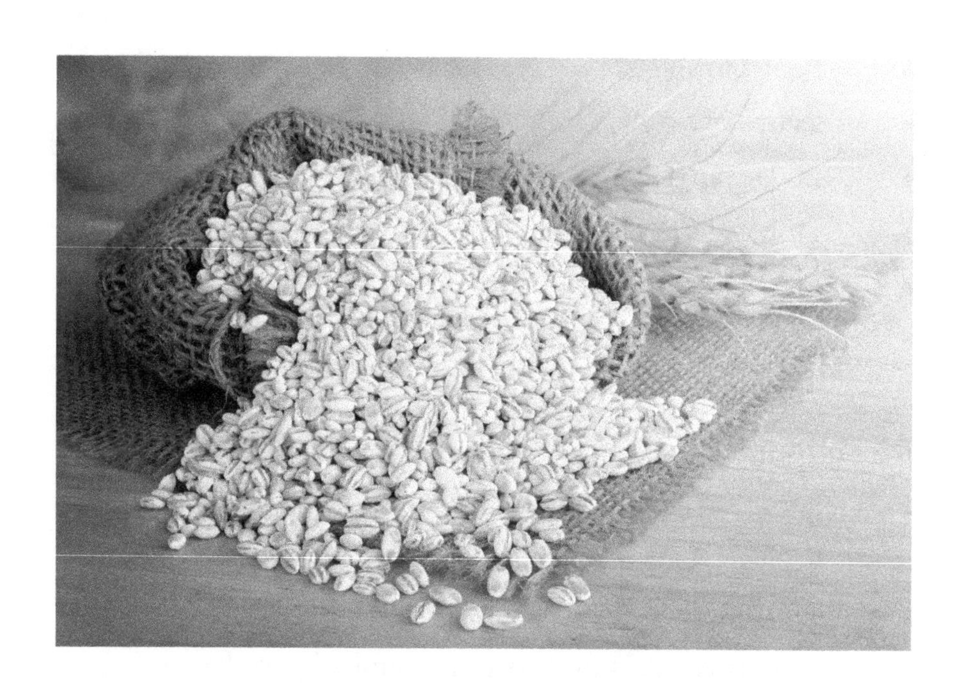

Creamed Corn

Prep time: 8 minutes Cooking time: 9 minutes Servings: 3

Ingredients:

- 2 cups frozen corn
- 1 cup vegetable broth
- ½ teaspoon salt
- 1 teaspoon yeast
- 1 cup coconut cream
- ½ teaspoon turmeric
- ½ teaspoon chili flakes

Directions:

10. In the mixing bowl whisk together vegetable broth, salt, yeast, coconut cream, turmeric, and chili flakes.
11. Place frozen corn in the instant pot bowl.
12. Pour coconut cream mixture over the corn and close the lid.
13. Set Manual mode (High pressure) and cook it for 9 minutes. Use quick pressure release.

Nutrition value/serving: calories 290, fat 20.8, fiber 4.9, carbs 24.8, protein 7.3

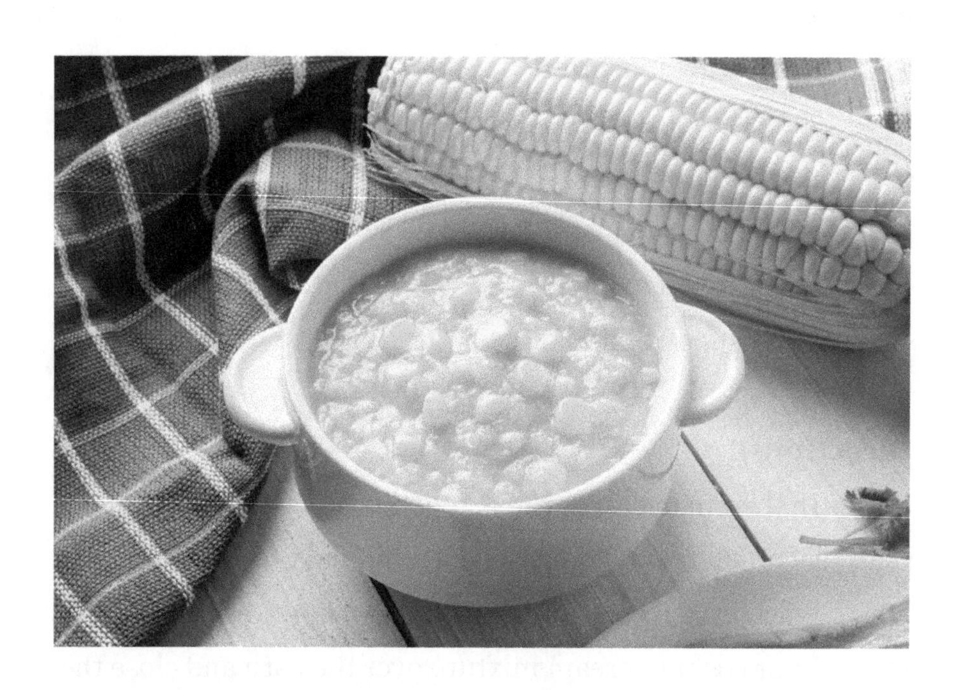

Mac’n Cheese

Prep time: 10 minutes Cooking time: 7 minutes Servings: 4

Ingredients:

- 2 cups macaroni
- 1 cup of water
- ½ cup cashew milk
- 1 teaspoon salt
- 5 oz vegan Parmesan, grated
- 1 teaspoon olive oil
- ½ teaspoon paprika

Directions:

11. Pour water in the instant pot. Add macaroni and salt. Close the lid.
12. Set Manual mode (High pressure) and cook the mixture for 3 minutes. Then use quick pressure release.
13. Drain the water from macaroni and return it back in the instant pot bowl.
14. Add cashew milk, olive oil, paprika, and grated Parmesan. Mix up the meal.
15. Close the lid and set Saute mode for 4 minutes.

16. When the meal is cooked – all the cheese should melt. Mix it up carefully before serving.

Nutrition value/serving: calories 278, fat 2.1, fiber 1.4, carbs 38.9, protein 20

Green Beans with Nuts

Prep time: 8 minutes Cooking time: 5 minutes Servings: 4

Ingredients:

- 2 cups green beans
- 1 teaspoon salt
- 2 cups vegetable broth
- 1 tablespoon olive oil
- ½ teaspoon garlic powder
- ¼ cup walnuts, chopped

Directions:

10. Set Saute mode and toss green beans in the instant pot.
11. Saute the vegetables for 2-3 minutes. Stir them from time to time.
12. Then add vegetable broth and close the lid.
13. Set Manual mode (High pressure) and cook the meal for 1 minute. Then use quick pressure release.
14. Drain vegetable broth and sprinkle vegetables with garlic powder and walnuts. Shake well and close the lid.
15. Saute the meal for 2-3 minutes more.

Nutrition value/serving: calories 116, fat 8.9, fiber 2.4, carbs 5.4, protein 5.4

Potato Salad

Prep time: 15 minutes Cooking time: 6 minutes Servings: 4

Ingredients:

- 3 red potatoes, peeled, chopped
- 1 cup green peas, frozen
- 1 tablespoon vegan mayonnaise
- 1 teaspoon mustard
- ½ teaspoon paprika
- 3 tablespoons fresh dill, chopped
- 2 tablespoons fresh parsley, chopped
- 1 teaspoon salt
- 1 cup water, for cooking

Directions:

10. Pour water in instant pot and insert steamer rack.
11. Place potatoes in the instant pot pan and transfer it in the instant pot.
12. Close the lid and cook the vegetables on Manual (High pressure) for 6 minutes.
13. After this, allow natural pressure release for 5 minutes.
14. Transfer the cooked potatoes in the salad bowl.

15. Then return back the pan in the instant pot and add frozen green peas.

16. Close the lid and cook them on Manual (High pressure) for 1 minute. Use quick pressure release.

17. Transfer the green peas in the salad bowl.

18. Add fresh dill and parsley.

19. In the separate small bowl whisk together paprika, mustard, salt, and vegan mayonnaise.

20. Pour the sauce over the salad mixture and mix up well.

Nutrition value/serving: calories 161, fat 1.6, fiber 5.2, carbs 32.7, protein 5.8

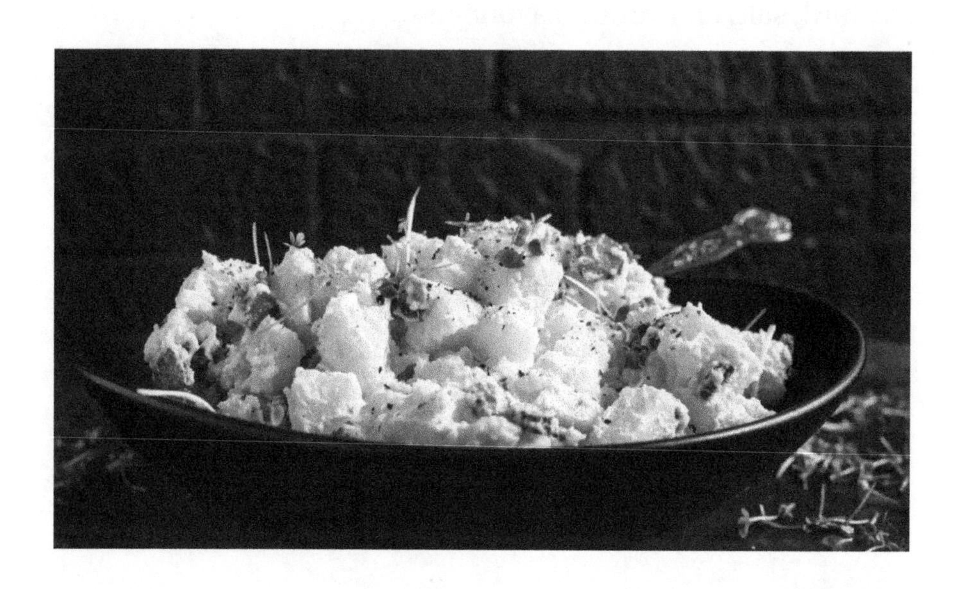

Cilantro Brussel Sprouts

Prep time: 5 minutes Cooking time: 4 minutes Servings: 2

Ingredients:

- 1 cup Brussel sprouts
- 1 garlic clove, peeled
- ½ cup of water
- 1 tablespoon dried cilantro
- ½ teaspoon salt
- 1 tablespoon olive oil

Directions:

9. Pour water and add Brussel sprouts in the instant pot.
10. Close the lid and cook vegetables on High pressure for 2 minutes.
11. Then use quick pressure release and drain water.
12. Chop garlic and add in Brussel sprouts.
13. Then add dried cilantro, salt, and olive oil. Mix up the vegetables and saute on Saute mode for 2 minutes.

Nutrition value/serving: calories 81, fat 7.2, fiber 1.7, carbs 4.5, protein 1.6

Mushroom Risotto

Prep time: 10 minutes Cooking time: 12 minutes Servings: 4

Ingredients:

- 1 cup mushrooms, chopped
- 1 tablespoon olive oil
- 1 white onion, diced
- ½ cup green peas, frozen
- ½ teaspoon dried thyme
- 1 teaspoon salt
- 1 ½ cups of rice
- 1 teaspoon garlic powder
- 2 ½ cups vegetable broth
- 1 teaspoon dried parsley
- 1 oz vegan Parmesan, grated

Directions:

8. Preheat instant pot on Saute mode.
9. Add olive oil, mushrooms, and diced onion. Saute vegetables for 5 minutes. Stir time to time.
10. Then add green peas, dried thyme, salt, garlic powder, and dried parsley.
11. Mix up well and add rice.

12. Then add vegetable broth and mix up.

13. Close the lid and cook risotto on Manual mode (High pressure) and cook it for 7 minutes.

14. Then use quick pressure release.

15. Open the lid and add grated vegan Parmesan. Mix up well.

Nutrition value/serving: calories 361, fat 5, fiber 2.7, carbs 63.9, protein 12.8

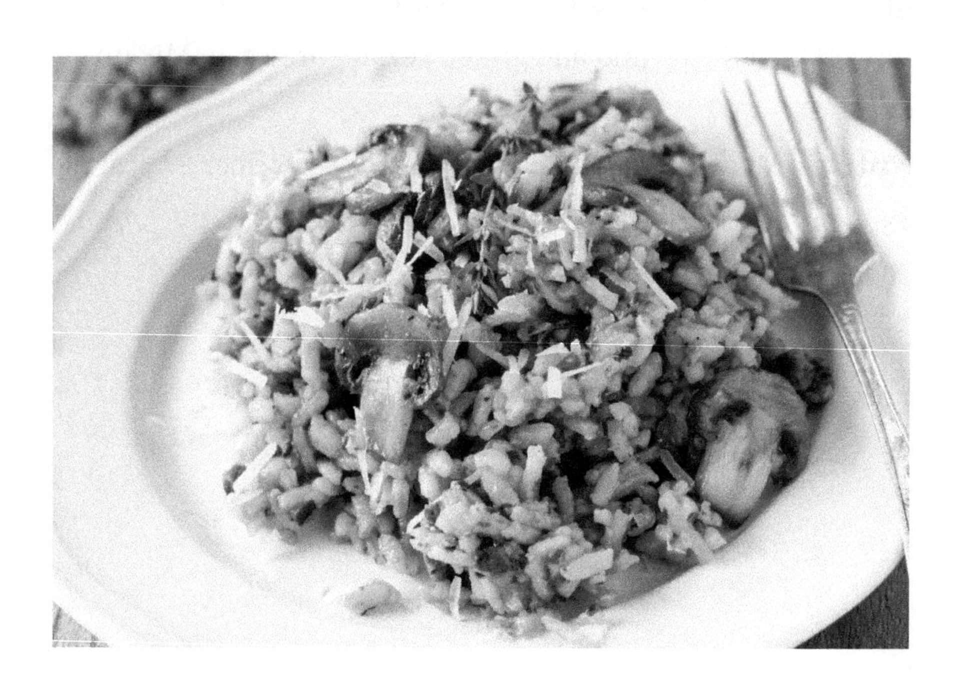

Ratatouille

Prep time: 10 minutes Cooking time: 15 minutes Servings: 6

Ingredients:

- 1 cup tomatoes, chopped
- 3 sweet peppers, chopped
- 1 red onion, diced
- 2 garlic cloves, peeled
- 1 zucchini, chopped
- ½ eggplant, chopped
- 2 tablespoons sesame oil
- 1 tablespoon fresh parsley, chopped
- 1 teaspoon tomato paste
- 1 teaspoon dried cilantro
- ¼ teaspoon dried oregano
- 1 tablespoon Italian seasoning
- 1 jalapeno, pepper, chopped
- 2 cups vegetable broth

Directions:

9. Set instant pot on Saute mode for 8 minutes and pour sesame oil.

10. Add sweet peppers, tomatoes, and onions. Stir the mixture.

11. Then add zucchini, garlic clove, eggplant, and jalapeno pepper.

12. Mix up the vegetables and keep cooking.

13. Add parsley, dried oregano, Italian seasoning, and tomato paste.

14. When the time of sauteing is over – add vegetable broth and close the lid.

15. Cook the meal on Manual mode (High pressure) for 2 minutes. Allow natural pressure release for 5 minutes.

Nutrition value/serving: calories 110, fat 6.1, fiber 3.4, carbs 12, protein 3.6

Pineapple Rice

Prep time: 5 minutes Cooking time: 8 minutes Servings: 4

Ingredients:

- 1 ½ cup of rice
- 2 cups of water
- 1 cup pineapple juice
- 1 can pineapples, chopped
- 1 teaspoon coconut cream

Directions:

10. Pour water and pineapple juice in the instant pot. Add rice and chopped pineapple, and close the lid.
11. Set Manual mode (high pressure) for 8 minutes. Then use quick pressure release.
12. Transfer the cooked pineapple rice in the bowl and add coconut cream. Stir it.

Nutrition value/serving: calories 310, fat 0.9, fiber 1.6, carbs 69, protein 5.4

Mongolian Stir Fry

Prep time: 5 minutes Cooking time: 4 minutes Servings: 4

Ingredients:

- 1 tablespoon minced ginger
- 1 teaspoon minced garlic
- 1 tablespoon avocado oil
- 4 tablespoons soy sauce
- 1 teaspoon chili flakes
- 1 teaspoon cornstarch
- 1 tablespoon brown sugar
- 8 tablespoon water
- ½ teaspoon cayenne pepper
- 1-pound seitan, chopped

Directions:

7. In the mixing bowl whisk together minced ginger, minced garlic, avocado oil, soy sauce, chili flakes, cornstarch, brown sugar, cayenne pepper, and water.
8. Preheat instant pot bowl on Saute mode until hot.
9. Transfer ginger mixture in the instant pot and cook it for 1 minute.
10. Then add chopped seitan and stir well.

11. Close the lid and set Manual mode (high pressure) for 1 minute. Use quick pressure release.
12. Mix up the side dish well before serving.

Nutrition value/serving: calories 59, fat 0.9, fiber 0.8, carbs 5.6, protein 6.6

Mushroom “Bacon”

Prep time: 5 minutes Cooking time: 2 minutes Servings: 5

Ingredients:

- 6 oz shiitake mushrooms
- 1 teaspoon salt
- ¼ teaspoon cayenne pepper
- 1 tablespoon olive oil

Directions:

5. Slice the mushrooms onto bacon shape strips and sprinkle every strip with olive oil, cayenne pepper, and salt.
6. Then place mushroom “bacon” in the instant pot and close the lid.
7. Set Manual mode (high pressure) and cook mushrooms for 2 minutes. Then use quick pressure release. The time of cooking depends on mushroom strips size.

Nutrition value/serving: calories 43, fat 2.9, fiber 0.7, carbs 4.7, protein 0.5

Crushed Baby Potatoes

Prep time: 10 minutes Cooking time: 10 minutes Servings: 2

Ingredients:

- 1 ½ cup baby potatoes
- 1 teaspoon salt
- 4 tablespoons olive oil
- 1 tablespoon dried rosemary
- 1 teaspoon dried oregano

Directions:

10. Wash baby potatoes carefully and crush with the help of the knife.
11. Then sprinkle the crushed potatoes with salt, olive oil, dried rosemary, and oregano.
12. Shake well until homogenous.
13. Transfer potatoes in the instant pot and close the lid.
14. Cook the meal on Manual mode (high pressure) for 4 minutes.
15. Then use natural pressure release for 5 minutes. Don't mix up potatoes anymore.

Nutrition value/serving: calories 325, fat 28.4, fiber 3.7, carbs 19.2, protein 2.1

Bang Bang Broccoli

Prep time: 10 minutes Cooking time: 4 minutes Servings: 2

Ingredients:

- 2 tablespoons vegan mayo
- 1 teaspoon chili paste
- 1 tablespoon Maple syrup
- 1 cup broccoli
- ¼ cup almond milk
- 1 teaspoon cornstarch
- 2 tablespoons wheat flour
- 1 teaspoon olive oil
- 1/3 cup panko bread crumbs
- 1 tablespoon lemon juice
- ½ cup water for cooking

Directions:

9. For the sauce: whisk together vegan mayo and chili paste.
10. For the broccoli batter: in the separated bowl whisk together almond milk, wheat flour, olive oil, cornstarch, and lemon juice.
11. Cut broccoli into the florets and dip into the batter.

12. Then coat every broccoli floret in the panko bread crumbs.

13. Pour water in the instant pot bowl and insert rack.

14. Place coated broccoli on the rack and close the lid.

15. Cook the vegetables on Manual mode (High pressure) for 4 minutes. Use quick pressure release.

16. Transfer the cooked broccoli in the bowl and sprinkle with sauce.

Nutrition value/serving: calories 280, fat 14.7, fiber 2.9, carbs 33.7, protein 5.4

Tikka Masala with Cauliflower

Prep time: 10 minutes Cooking time: 10 minutes Servings: 4

Ingredients:

- 1 teaspoon garam masala
- ½ teaspoon salt
- 1 cup cauliflower, chopped
- 1/3 cup coconut yogurt
- 1 teaspoon ground cumin
- ½ teaspoon ground coriander
- 1 onion, diced
- ½ teaspoon garlic, diced
- ¼ teaspoon minced ginger
- 1 cup tomatoes, canned

Directions:

6. Set instant pot on Saute mode.
7. Add olive oil, diced onion, garlic, and minced ginger.
8. Then sprinkle the mixture with ground cumin, coriander, salt, and garam masala.
9. Mix up well.
10. Add canned tomatoes and mix up well. Saute the mixture for 5 minutes.

11. After this, add chopped cauliflower and stir well.

12. Close the lid and seal it. Cook the meal on Manual mode (High pressure) for 3 minutes.

13. Then use quick pressure release and open the lid.

14. Add coconut yogurt and mix up well. Serve the meal hot

Nutrition value/serving: calories 67, fat 4.1, fiber 1.8, carbs 7.2, protein 1.7

Vegetable En Papillote

Prep time: 10 minutes Cooking time: 3 minutes Servings: 4

Ingredients:

- 1 cup baby carrot
- ½ cup green beans
- 1 teaspoon dried rosemary
- 1 teaspoon salt
- 1 tablespoon avocado oil
- 1 garlic clove, diced
- 1 teaspoon fresh oregano
- 1 tablespoon lemon juice
- 1 teaspoon turmeric

Directions:

9. In the mixing bowl mix up together baby carrot and green beans.
10. Sprinkle the vegetables with dried rosemary, salt, avocado oil, garlic, oregano, lemon juice, and turmeric. Shake the ingredients well.
11. Then Wrap the vegetables in the baking paper and transfer in the instant pot.
12. Close the lid and seal it.

13. Cook the vegetables on Manual mode (High pressure) for 3 minutes.

14. Then allow natural pressure release for 5 minutes and remove vegetables from the baking paper.

Nutrition value/serving: calories 30, fat 0.7, fiber 2.3, carbs 5.8, protein 0.7

Brown Rice

Prep time: 15 minutes Cooking time: 18 minutes Servings: 4

Ingredients:

- 1 ½ cup brown rice
- 3 cups of water
- 1 tablespoon olive oil
- 1 teaspoon salt

Directions:

7. Set Saute mode and preheat instant pot.
8. Add olive oil and brown rice and stir it well.
9. Cook the rice for 3 minutes.
10. Add water and salt. Close and seal the lid.
11. Set Manual mode (high pressure) and cook the meal for 15 minutes.
12. Allow natural pressure release for 10 minutes more.
13. Mix up the rice before serving.

Nutrition value/serving: calories 57, fat 3.9, fiber 0, carbs 5.3, protein 0.4

Fragrant Bulgur

Prep time: 5 minutes Cooking time: 19 minutes Servings: 3

Ingredients:

- 1 cup bulgur
- 1 teaspoon tomato paste
- 2 cup of water
- 1 teaspoon olive oil
- 1 teaspoon salt

Directions:

6. Preheat instant pot on Saute mode and add olive oil.
7. Place bulgur in the oil and stir well. Saute it for 4 minutes.
8. Then add tomato paste and salt. Stir well.
9. Add water and mix up bulgur until you get a homogenous liquid mixture.
10. Close the lid and set Manual mode (low pressure).
11. Cook bulgur for 15 minutes.
12. The bulgur will be cooked when it soaks all the liquid.

Nutrition value/serving: calories 174, fat 2.2, fiber 8.6, carbs 35.8, protein 5.8

Baked Apples

Prep time: 5 minutes Cooking time: 9 minutes Servings: 6

Ingredients:

- 4 red apples, chopped
- 1 teaspoon ground cinnamon
- 1 tablespoon brown sugar
- 1 teaspoon maple syrup
- ¼ cup cashew milk

Directions:

8. Place apples in the instant pot and sprinkle with ground cinnamon, brown sugar, and maple syrup.
9. Close the lid and set Saute mode. Cook the apples for 5 minutes.
10. Then add cashew milk and mix up the side dish well.
11. Cook it for 4 minutes more.

Nutrition value/serving: calories 88, fat 0.4, fiber 3.8, carbs 23.1, protein 0.4

Scalloped Potatoes

Prep time: 15 minutes Cooking time: 4 minutes Servings: 4

Ingredients:

- 4 potatoes, peeled, sliced
- 1 cup almond milk
- 1 teaspoon nutritional yeast
- 1 teaspoon dried rosemary
- ½ teaspoon salt
- 1 teaspoon garlic powder
- 1 teaspoon cashew butter
- 1 teaspoon ground nutmeg

Directions:

8. Mix up together nutritional yeast, dried rosemary, salt, garlic powder, and ground nutmeg. Whisk together almond milk and spice mixture.
9. Grease the instant pot bowl with cashew butter.
10. Place the sliced potatoes inside instant pot bowl by layers.
11. Then pour almond milk mixture over the potatoes and close the lid.

12. Cook scalloped potatoes on Manual mode (High pressure) for 4 minutes. Then allow natural pressure release for 10 minutes.

13. Sprinkle the cooked meal with your favorite vegan cheese if desired.

Nutrition value/serving: calories 302, fat 15.5, fiber 7, carbs 38.5, protein 5.7

Glazed White Onions

Prep time: 5 minutes Cooking time: 20 minutes Servings: 4

Ingredients:

- 3 white onions, peeled, sliced
- 1 tablespoon sugar
- ½ teaspoon ground black pepper
- 3 tablespoons coconut oil
- ½ teaspoon baking soda

Directions:

7. Set Saute mode and preheat instant pot until hot.
8. Toss coconut oil and melt it.
9. When the coconut oil is liquid, add sugar, baking soda, and ground black pepper. Stir the mixture gently.
10. Add sliced onions and mix the ingredients up.
11. Close the lid and saute onions for 15 minutes.
12. When the side dish is cooked it will have a light brown color and tender texture.

Nutrition value/serving: calories 133, fat 10.3, fiber 1.8, carbs 10.9, protein 0.9

Spicy Garlic

Prep time: 10 minutes Cooking time: 10 minutes Servings: 4

Ingredients:

- 4 garlic bulbs, trimmed
- 2 teaspoons olive oil
- ½ teaspoon salt
- ¼ teaspoon chili flakes
- ½ cup water, for cooking

Directions:

7. Pour water in the instant pot and insert rack.
8. Place garlic bulbs on the rack and sprinkle with olive oil, salt, and chili flakes.
9. Close the lid and set Poultry mode.
10. Cook garlic for 10 minutes. Then allow natural pressure release for 5 minutes more.
11. Serve the garlic when it reaches room temperature.

Nutrition value/serving: calories 35, fat 2.3, fiber 0, carbs 3, protein 0

Pasta and Green Peas Side Dish

Prep time: 5 minutes Cooking time: 10 minutes Servings: 2

Ingredients:

- ½ cup pasta
- 1 cup of water
- 1/3 cup green peas, frozen
- 1 teaspoon salt
- ¼ teaspoon minced garlic
- 1 teaspoon tomato paste

Directions:

6. Mx up together water, tomato paste, minced garlic, and salt.
7. Pout liquid in the instant pot. Add green peas and pasta. Mix up gently.
8. Close the lid and set Manual mode (High pressure).
9. Cook the side dish for 10 minutes. Then use quick pressure release.
10. Drain ½ part of the liquid and transfer the meal into the serving bowl.s

Nutrition value/serving: calories 207, fat 1.6, fiber 1.4, carbs 39.1, protein 8.7

Almond Milk Millet

Prep time: 5 minutes Cooking time: 10 minutes Servings: 3

Ingredients:

- ½ teaspoon salt
- 1 cup millet
- 1 cup almond milk

Directions:

11. Pour almond milk in the instant pot bowl.
12. Add millet and salt.
13. Close and seal the lid and set Manual mode (High pressure).
14. Cook the side dish for 10 minutes. Allow natural pressure release.

Nutrition value/serving: calories 436, fat 21.9, fiber 7.4, carbs 53, protein 9.2

Stir Fried Kale

Prep time: 5 minutes Cooking time: 5 minutes Servings: 4

Ingredients:

- 2 cup kale, chopped
- ½ teaspoon nutritional yeast
- 1 teaspoon coconut oil
- ½ teaspoon ground black pepper
- 2 tablespoon bread crumbs
- 4 tablespoons water

Directions:

6. Preheat instant pot on Saute mode until hot.
7. Toss coconut oil and melt it.
8. Add chopped kale and sprinkle it with ground black pepper and nutritional yeast.
9. Add water and saute kale for 2 minutes.
10. Then mix up kale well and sprinkle with bread crumbs.
11. Close the lid and cook on Manual mode (high pressure) for 1 minute. Allow quick pressure release.
12. Shake the kale well before serving.

Nutrition value/serving: calories 42, fat 1.3, fiber 0.8, carbs 6.3, protein 1.7

Zoodles

Prep time: 10 minutes Cooking time: 25 minutes Servings: 4

Ingredients:

- 2 zucchini
- ½ teaspoon salt
- ¾ cup vegetable broth
- ¼ teaspoon ground black pepper

Directions:

11. Wash and trim zucchini well.
12. With the help of the spiralizer make the zucchini zoodles.
13. Sprinkle them with ground black pepper and salt.
14. Transfer zoodles in the instant pot bowl and add vegetable broth.
15. Close and seal the lid. Set Manual moe (high pressure) and cook meal for 1 minute. Use natural pressure release.

Nutrition value/serving: calories 23, fat 0.4, fiber 1.1, carbs 3.5, protein 2.1

Buckwheat

Prep time: 10 minutes Cooking time: 15 minutes Servings: 4

Ingredients:

- 2 cups buckwheat
- 2.5 cup of water
- 1 tablespoon sunflower oil
- 1 teaspoon salt
- 1 tablespoon almond butter

Directions:

1. Pour sunflower oil in the instant pot. Add almond butter and saute the ingredients for 3 minutes on Saute mode.
2. Then add buckwheat and stir it carefully. Saute the mixture for 3 minutes.
3. Add water and stir well.
4. Close and seal the lid.
5. Set manual mode (high pressure) and cook buckwheat for 4 minutes.
6. Then use quick pressure release.
7. Mix up the buckwheat carefully before serving.

Nutrition value/serving: calories 347, fat 8.6, fiber 8.9, carbs 61.5, protein 12.1

CPSIA information can be obtained
at www.ICGtesting.com
Printed in the USA
BVHW061412250221
601119BV00001B/122